Fall 2020

HOPE

Brain Injury
HOPE
MAGAZINE
*"Supporting the
Brain Injury Community"*

Welcome

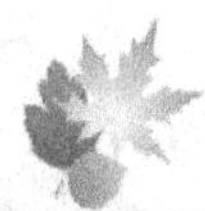

HOPE MAGAZINE

Serving the Brain Injury Community Since 2015

Fall 2020

Publisher
David A. Grant

Editor
Sarah Grant

Our Contributors
Stacia Bissell
Patrick Brigham
William Carter
Eddie Conrardy
Andrew Davie
Jen Dodge
Sarah V. Jackson
Roman Ponomarchuks
Thomas Sanders
James Scott
Lyrsa Smith
Samantha Stachulski
Rebecca Veenstra

Welcome to the Fall 2020 Issue of HOPE Magazine

Since the publication of the first issue of HOPE Magazine back in 2015, our core mission remains unchanged: *To bring to our readership a diverse range of stories that reflect brain injury as it really is.*

Sometimes this means delving into tough topics, but to offer anything less than what amounts to the true reality of life after brain injury would be to disserve our readership.

Yet among all the challenges remains what is our most powerful message – there is real and meaningful hope abounding in today's troubled world.

This month's issue features stories from brain injury survivors, spouses, and family members alike. Our first story, submitted by a younger contributor, speaks of what it is like growing up in a home with a brain injured parent.

A wonderful article, it is also the first time that we have had a father/daughter team of contributors, as we have published her dad's writing several times over the years. Thank you Samantha, for your courage in sharing your truths.

Be safe and be kind.

Peace,

David A. Grant
Publisher

Table of Contents

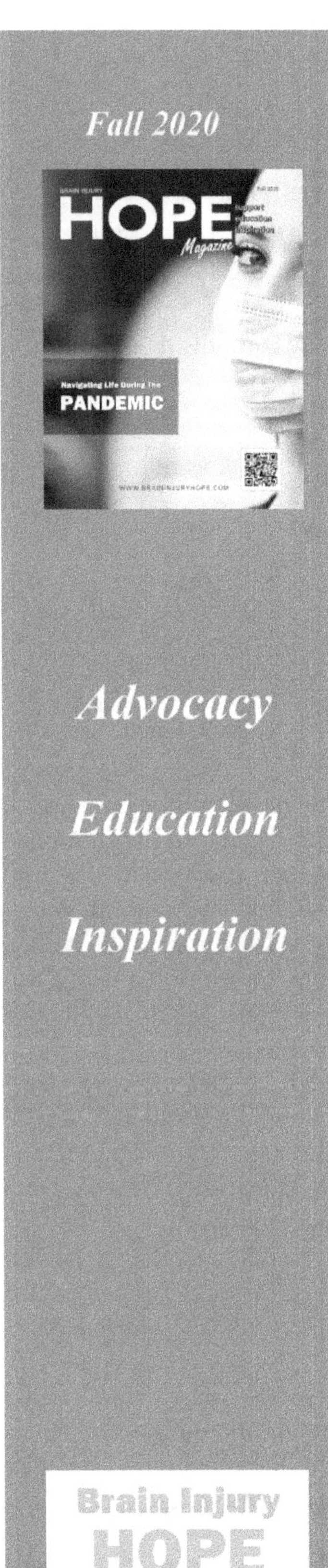

Discovering Me

By Samantha Stachulski

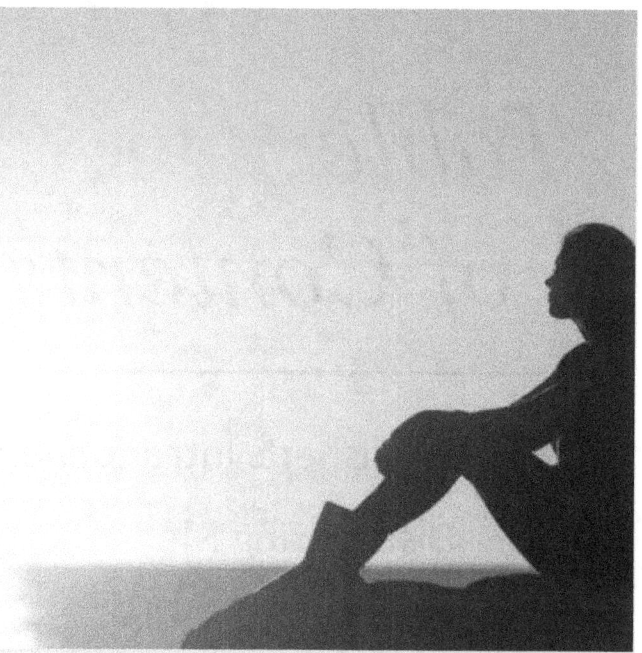

My name is Samantha Stachulski, and I am the daughter of a Traumatic Brain Injury Survivor. Shortly before I was born, my father was severely injured in a motor vehicle accident which, *in an instant*, changed his life forever. As a child, I watched him suffer tremendously with many physical, cognitive, behavioral, and psychosocial problems.

Because stigma prevented him from asking anyone for help, he struggled for many years to perform several activities of daily living and his job.

After my parents separated, my father finally agreed to get medical help at a local VA hospital. With the help of many doctors and therapists, he began the long and slow process of learning strategies that would improve the quality of his life and the lives of his family members. Through it all, my family became resilient, empathetic, and grateful, and we learned how to achieve our goals through hard work and perseverance. Against all odds, my parents stayed together, and we worked together to advocate for others whose lives had been affected by a brain injury.

> *"It wasn't easy being the child of a disabled parent. It was very scary, lonely, embarrassing, hopeless, and traumatic for me."*

It wasn't easy being the child of a disabled parent. It was very scary, lonely, embarrassing, hopeless, and traumatic for me. My father's disability often overshadowed who I was and my abilities. I often felt like I had no voice and was invisible. To help me overcome the many odds stacked against me, my father said to me, "It's better to be well rounded than to be the best at only 1 thing!"

I believe this was his way of letting me know that I'm my own person and to encourage me to follow all of my dreams and achieve all of my goals. This is when my father's disability stopped overshadowing me and my own story of *hope and inspiration* began.

I wasn't the best youth softball player, but I worked hard to learn how to play the game. I played any position my coaches needed me to play without complaining. My hard work and good sportsmanship helped me become a very productive teammate on two championship teams.

I'm not the best hip hop or jazz dancer, but for the past eight years I've shown up to practices and stayed after to learn the dance routines. Even though I'm the girl in the back trying hard not to look awkward, I make my dance mates, instructors, and parents very proud by performing well at my dance recitals.

I'm not the best student, but I work extra hard late into the night to fill my brain with knowledge. My teachers respect me because I participate fully in class, ask questions, and help other students. I'm participating in a Health Science Technology program and hope to obtain my Nursing Assistant License after I complete the course and pass the State licensing exam.

After COVID-19 hit, and my community was in a panic, I volunteered to increase my hours at the grocery store I work at as a way to help my community. Recently, I was promoted to work in the courtesy booth because the grocery store managers knew they could depend on me to help worried customers weather the storm and sea of unknowns the pandemic had brought to them.

Through my own struggles, I've risen up to become a well-rounded rock and a pillar to my family, classmates, teammates, coworkers, and community. I am resilient, empathetic, grateful, and a hard worker. I'm someone people can trust, rely upon, and call, "friend."

> **Through my own struggles, I've risen up to become a well-rounded rock and a pillar to my family, classmates, teammates, coworkers, and community.**

While I was *discovering me*, I still managed to fully participate in my local Brain Injury Community.

After I graduate high school, I plan on pursuing a college degree in Occupational Therapy. After Grad School, my goal is to treat people who have become injured, ill, or disabled, with the purpose of helping them regain their functioning and independence to improve their quality of life.

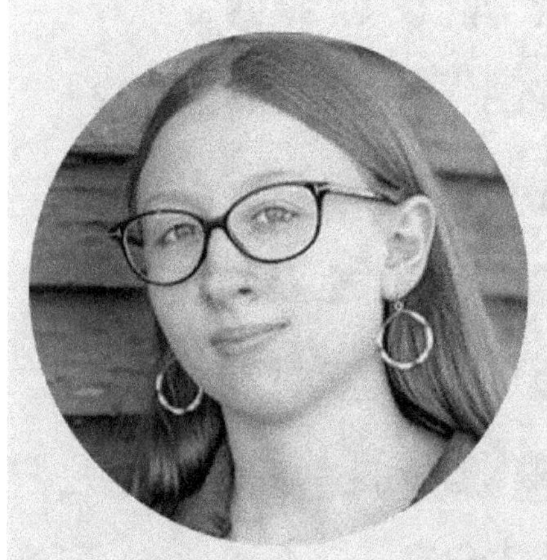

Samantha Stachulski

Samantha is a Senior at Timberlane Regional High School in Plaistow, New Hampshire. She is a brain injury advocate who has participated in many Brain Injury Association events and support groups. After graduating high school, Sam plans on pursuing a college degree in Occupational Therapy. After Grad School, her goal is to treat people who have become injured, ill, or disabled, with the purpose of helping them regain their functioning and independence and improve their quality of life.

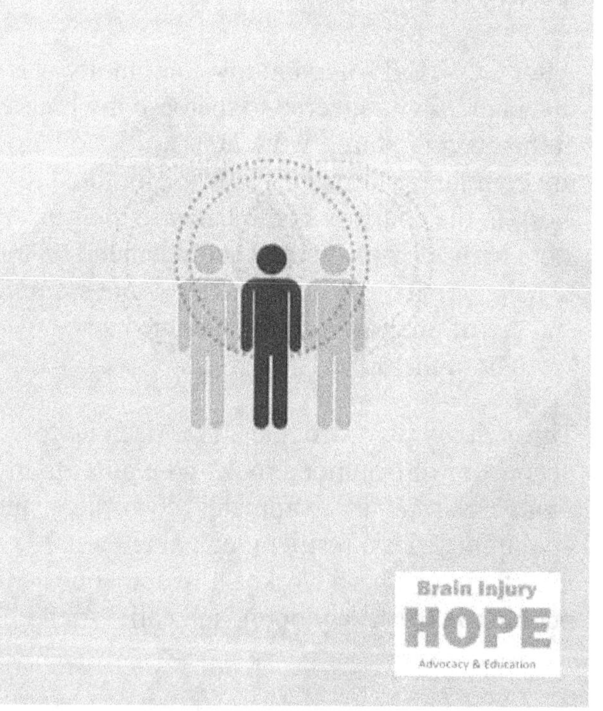

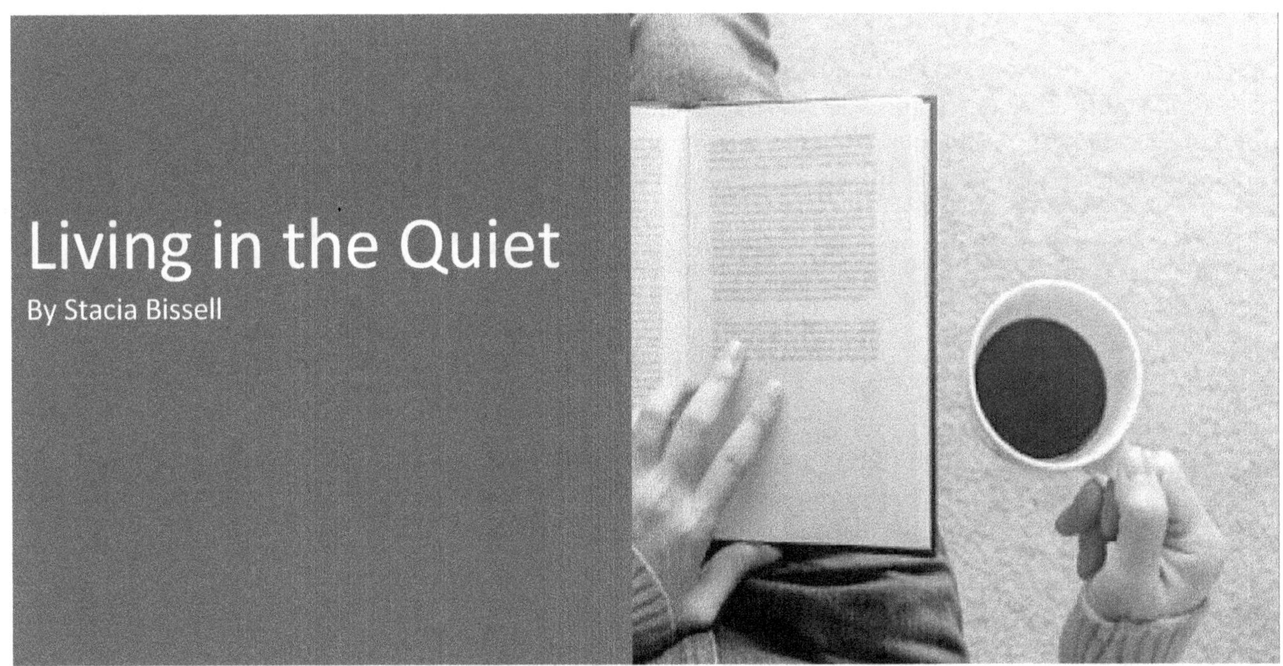

Living in the Quiet

By Stacia Bissell

It was the sudden departure from my job and then my divorce, both on the heels of my TBI that put a lid on my life as I knew it. It was the embarrassment of being broken in the brain *and* feeling like a failure as a wife *and* feeling the awkwardness of no longer being a well-known, successful and upstanding educator in my community that resulted in me questionably surviving in a world unrecognizable to me.

All of this is what kept me alone at home with a perpetual and painful case of FOMO *(Fear Of Missing Out)*. When you add in what social media told me was going on "out there," my case of FOMO seemed to get ten times worse.

Since walking away from my career in 2014 due to the high demands of my job as a middle school educator and the negative effect my job was having on my health due to a bicycle accident that resulted in a life-altering traumatic brain injury, the FOMO factor within me had been strong, depressing and anxiety-ridden. My social life literally came to a screeching halt half a decade ago.

> *"I would dread each Friday and Saturday night, knowing I would feel the familiar pull to be heading out the door to enjoy some restaurant or someone's home for a dinner party."*

I would dread each Friday and Saturday night, knowing I would feel the familiar pull to be heading out the door to enjoy some restaurant, someone's home for a dinner party, some music or theater venue, a bar, or a craft brewery. The reality was that I wouldn't be going anywhere. Before my TBI occurred, which just about coincides with me having an empty nest and being separated from my husband, he and I would always have plans on the weekends with at least two other people, if not six.

Since then, I have had nowhere to go, no work group to go with, no consistent special someone to go with - especially someone who understood my limitations and could get me out of a too-loud place quickly or see that I was fading and make a gracious excuse for an early departure. I felt like I had nothing to contribute anymore by way of interesting conversation anyway.

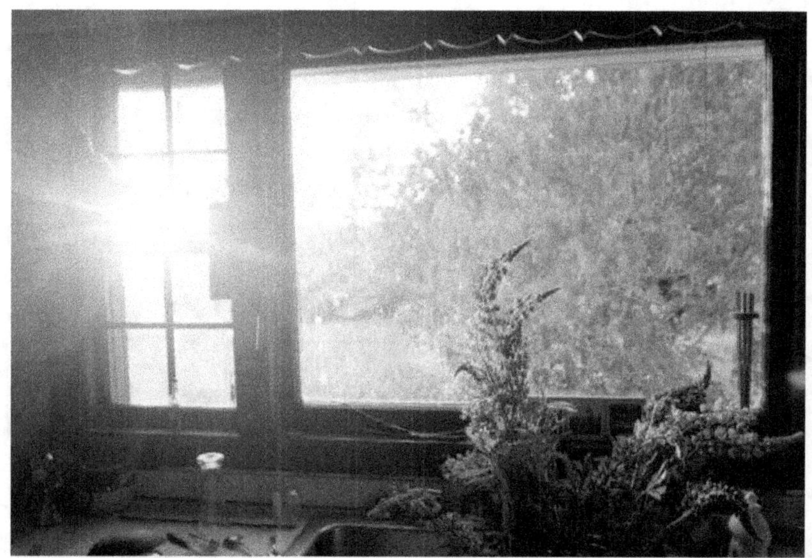

Now that almost everyone is home due to COVID restrictions, and I hear frequent grumbles about what people are missing out on and the struggle they are having associated with those losses, I actually feel I'm ahead of the curve again like I used to feel when I was my pre-TBI self. I had already adjusted to *living life in the quiet*, which can take a long, long time to get accustomed to for a number of reasons.

It is not going to happen in four or five months, I assure you. I had already learned how to be in my home for long periods of time without tearing my hair out. I know how to keep myself busy enough with never ending piles of photos to go through, closets to organize, gardens to expand, walls to paint, and recipes to try. I can use technology to stay in touch with those I care about. I can choose when and how to socialize distantly with dear ones at a local park or someone's deck or driveway and still feel COVID safe and secure.

My friends and family have embraced the BYOE model (*bring your own everything* - from chairs to beverages to food), so it's easier to get together *and* it releases me of any concerns over how to feed people. I am overjoyed to be able to keep up with conversations that smaller numbers of people offer me with my new, post-TBI auditory processing disorder.

I can choose to stay in my pajamas for hours in the morning without the fear of my doorbell ringing. I am not the holiday entertaining machine for my family and friends anymore, and therefore there is a sense of really living & relaxing in my home without constantly keeping my pantry stocked and every corner of every room cleaned and polished. This is working just fine for me. I feel like I am with the in crowd now. I feel calmer.

Personally, while I miss hugging my parents who are now 86 and 92, and having Sunday dinners with my 85 year-old Aunt, my own views have happily shifted away from FOMO.

> **I can choose to stay in my pajamas for hours in the morning without the fear of my doorbell ringing.**

I must admit that for the first time in years, I am actually pretty content that I'm sticking close to home. I guess you can say that I now fall into the JOMO category (*The Joy Of Missing Out*).

I'm seeing the glass half full and doing a silly little JOMO jig in my living room. No one will see me anyway.

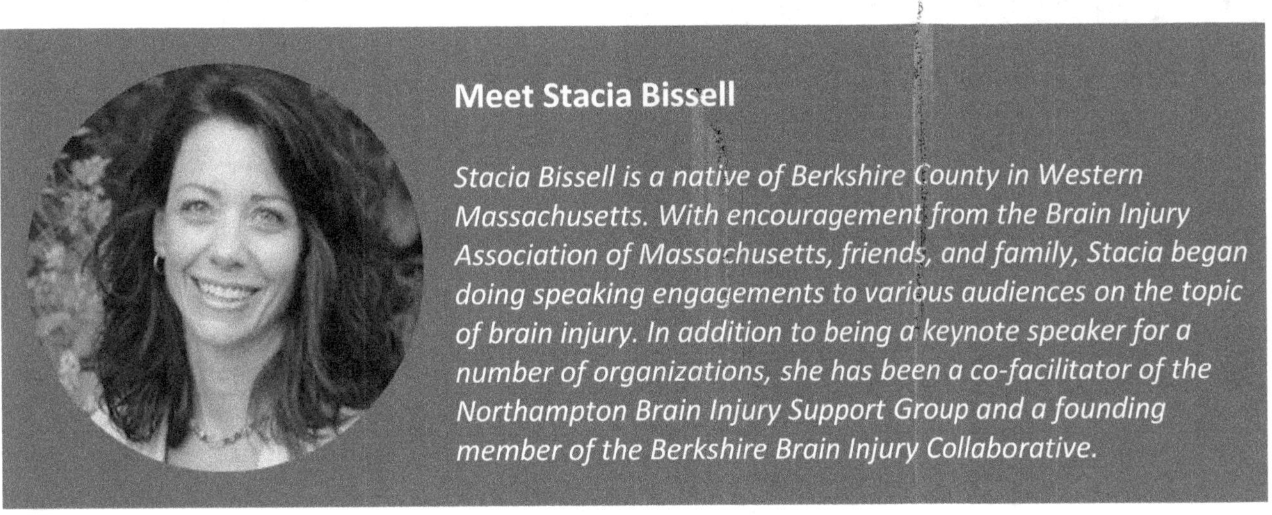

Meet Stacia Bissell

Stacia Bissell is a native of Berkshire County in Western Massachusetts. With encouragement from the Brain Injury Association of Massachusetts, friends, and family, Stacia began doing speaking engagements to various audiences on the topic of brain injury. In addition to being a keynote speaker for a number of organizations, she has been a co-facilitator of the Northampton Brain Injury Support Group and a founding member of the Berkshire Brain Injury Collaborative.

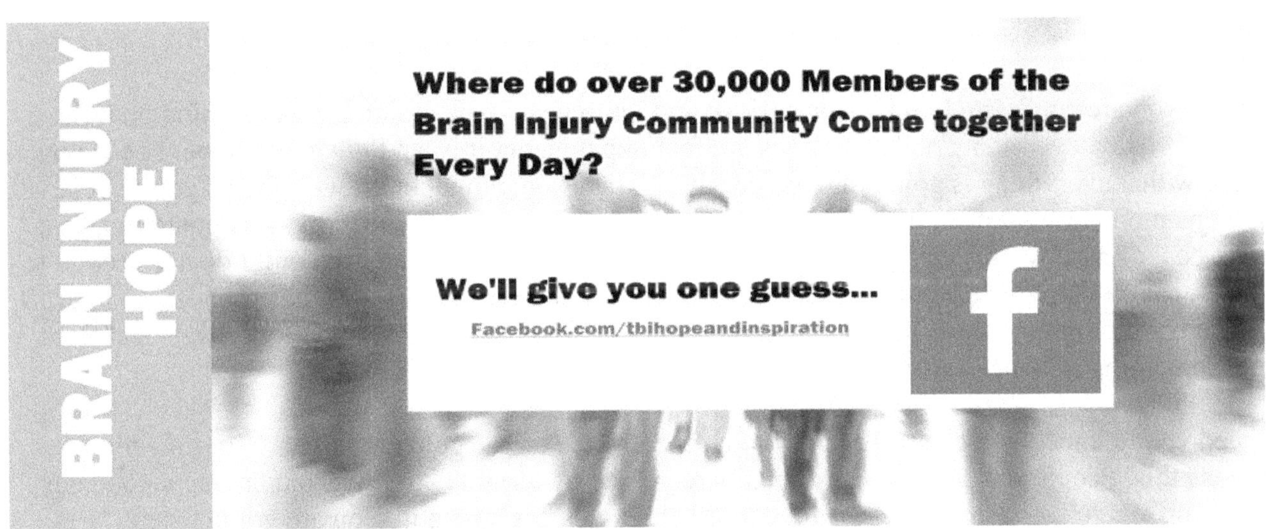

"Hope lies in dreams, in imagination, and in the courage of those who dare to make dreams into reality."

– Jonas Salk

Letter to the Newly Brain-Injured Me

By William Carter

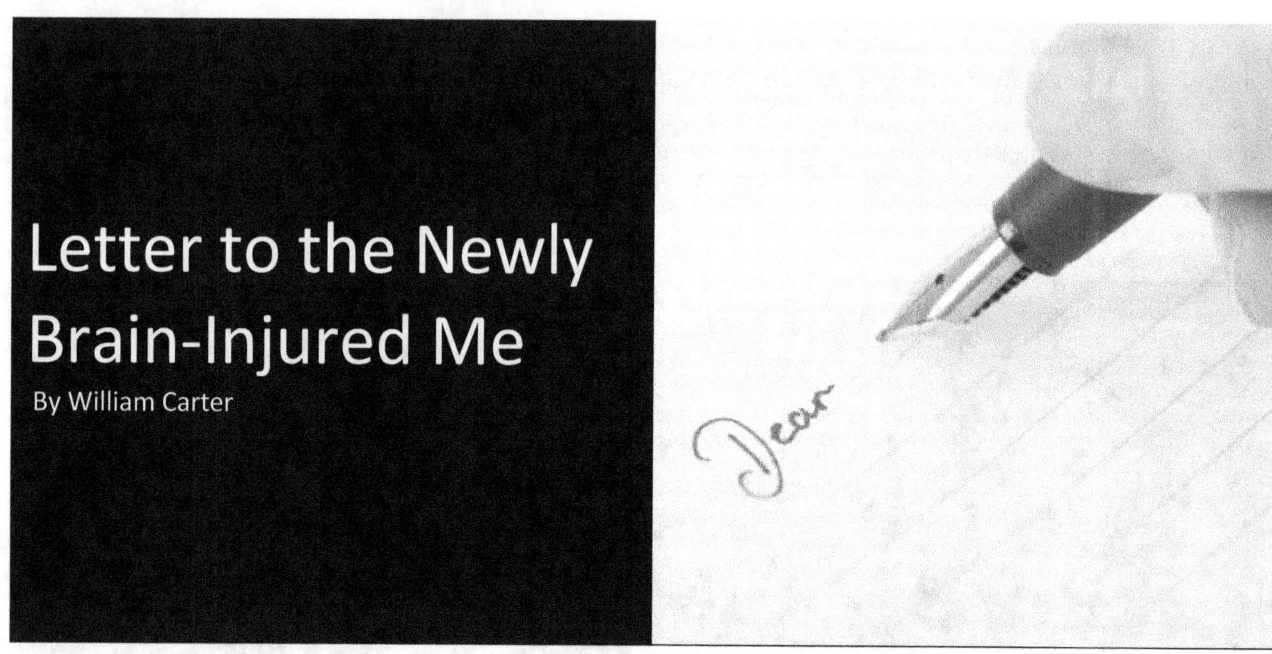

I invite you to read the letter that I wish the me of today could send the me who just woke up from a coma.

Dear Will,

I know you are confused. I know you are lost, and I know you have no idea what is going on right now. It's okay, everything's okay. It does not feel like it is, but it is, and it's going to be. I need you to know that everything is going to work out. It will take some time, but it will. I need you to believe that this moment right now, this moment you are in is going to take some work. It is going to take a great deal of hard work, determination, and you can get through it. Really though, I do not need to tell you that. You don't have a problem putting your nose to the grindstone - you never have. You have a problem with thinking the grindstone will fix things, that you can put enough blood sweat and tears into something to make it work.

I need you to understand that is it's okay to not be okay. You are going to have a hard time telling anyone this. People will naturally ask you, "Are you doing alright?" or "Are you having a good day?" And, you are going to smile because love it or hate it, you can't help it. You are going to say, "I'm doing great!" Though, you are not doing great. You are going to say you are, and some days, you're going to say it so much that, on those days, you're going to believe it. Stay in those moments. Rest in those moments where you feel okay but remember- promise me you are going to remember- that it's okay to not be okay.

Because, truth is, you are going to feel like a failure. Many times, over the next several years, you are going to feel like a wasted and squandered soul. There are times when your best is not going to be good enough. Remember that grindstone? You are going to break your nose on it, and you'll feel broken yourself. This is okay. Remember, things are going to work out.

"Every failure you experience, every mistake, missed opportunity, everything is not only a learning opportunity, it is a path towards where you need to be."

You are going to fall. Do not be afraid of it though. I know, you struggle with that, because you feel that, every time you fall, people think it is because of your disability. Forget them. People will put you in a box whether you like it or not. Show them their box is a failed exercise by shattering it, by learning from your failure and becoming something beautiful. Other people do not control you. Do not let your fear of what they might think stifle who you are.

Every failure you experience, every mistake, missed opportunity, everything is not only a learning opportunity, it is a path towards where you need to be. Failure is good. Stop hating your failure and embrace it. You messed up? Good. Where is that taking you? You are struggling? Good. Learn your place beyond the struggle. I know that they all sound like platitudes, but hear me Will, you are not a measure of your achievements, you are not your grades, you are not your friends, and you are not what others think of you. Now, this one will come much later, but you are not your paycheck.

If you never step off the ledge, you will never fly. If you let your fear of fulfilling the expectations you think people have for you, you will prove them right. Risk yields reward.

LIVE YOUR LIFE. SCREW UP.

Samuel Beckett once wrote, "Fail. Fail again. Fail better."

Now, I know you love Mr. Beckett, but he is wrong here. Fail. Fail again, but you can't be focused on failing better, you must be focused on seizing the opportunity, and learning from not just for the craft of writing, a specific activity or ability, but seizing the blessing the failure yields you. Failing better means trying the same thing again. Sometimes, that failure is to show you to do something differently, something new. Your failures in life are going to redirect you. Sometimes, those mistakes will point your life to something else.

You are going to feel like a failure in graduate school and that is okay. God is teaching you about where you need to be. Accept that. You are going to feel like a failure teaching high-school. Accept what you see as failure, and let it point you to the next thing. Make sure, though, to remember that no second of your life is wasted. Even in your "failures" you are being used.

Do not let your failures take away your shine. Let them direct where you need to point your light, but always make sure to breathe on the ember and make it shine brighter. You are healing. You are growing, and at any moment, any time, God is shaping you into who you will be and using you in the moments you cannot stand to be in and the moments you cannot enjoy who you are.

Your life is going to work out, trust me. Your failures? They will lead you to a beautiful woman who you will start a family with. And I know you - you want me to tell you your career will work out too. Right?

You are going to love what you do. You are going to fall, but everyone falls. You will have days where you feel like limp, smoldering wick, but all the while. Get out there. Live. Live and fail. Fall and tumble. Let your face be scratched and scarred, but even if you are missing a few teeth when you stand up, you are going to be smiling so broadly that you're not going to care.

> # Make sure, though, to remember that no second of your life is wasted. Even in your "failures" you are being used.

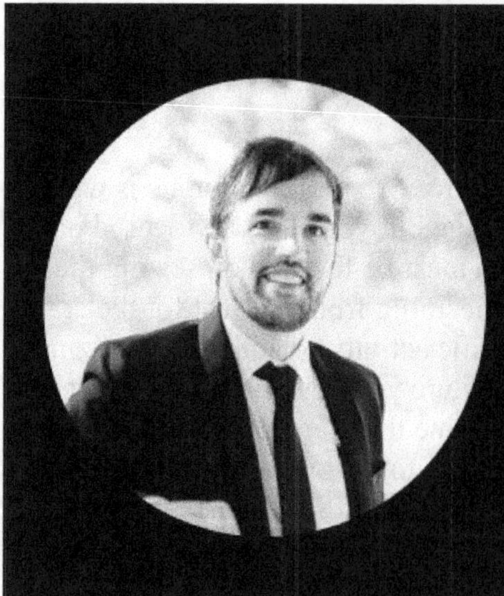

Meet William Carter

Will Carter is a native of Roswell, Georgia. He suffered a traumatic brain injury in October of 2007, while he was a senior at Roswell High School. After a stay at the Shepherd Center, he was blessed to go on to Oglethorpe University to receive his bachelor's degree in playwriting. From there, he went to Boston University to receive his M.F.A in Playwriting, and then, he went on to the University of Louisville to receive a master's degree in teaching. He loves his job, sharing his story with his students, and hoping to encourage and inspire them on to live their lives to the fullest.

Elvis Played the Cow Palace

By Andrew Davie

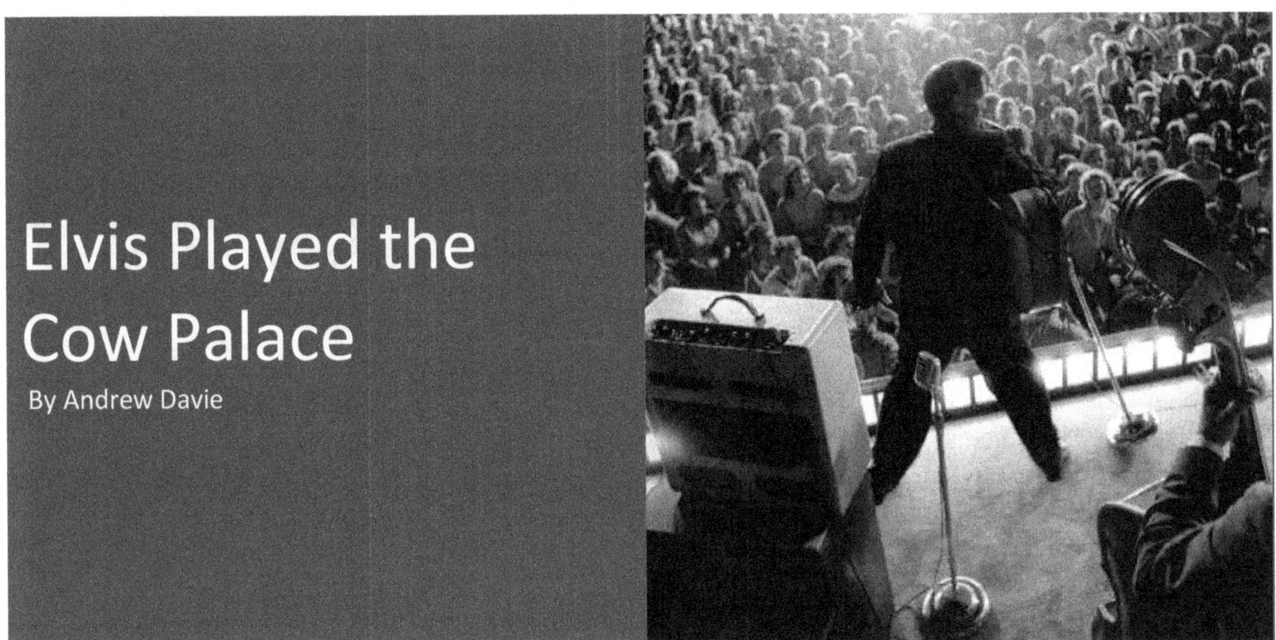

When I was in Graduate school, I wrote a short story entitled *"The Solitude of Fortress."* There had been a segment of the story I cut in which I discussed the movie Fortress starring Christopher Lambert. Kurtwood Smith from Robocop and later "That 70's Show" was in it, as well as Vernon Wells who played the mohawk-having villain Wez in *The Road Warrior,* The Lord General in Weird Science, and Bennett in Commando.

The title had been a play on words on Superman's Fortress of Solitude, but it was also a metaphor. There are very few people who are intimate with the details of the film Fortress. It can be a lonely existence. When I had my ruptured aneurysm, aside from a lengthy physical and emotional recovery, I also needed to figure out how I would spend my time.

> *"When I had my ruptured aneurysm, aside from a lengthy physical and emotional recovery, I also needed to figure out how I would spend my time."*

The goals I had had before the aneurysm had changed. As the months dragged on, I was plagued by existential ennui. Recently, I listened to a podcast that discussed theories Carl Jung and Friedrich Nietzsche had on the role mythology played in cultivating spiritual development and helping to provide comfort with the aforementioned question.

According to the show, one of the reasons people experience existential angst is due to the rise of technology eclipsing the role of mythology in our culture. "Myths are narratives which transmit modes of behavior, patterns of action, and ways of experiencing the world, that promote healthy psychological development and a meaningful life." -Academy of Ideas Podcast.

After my brain injury, the question of purpose reappeared. The analogy I think of is someone at the dinner table who is not hungry and has no tastebuds. Though they know they must eat, but it is also difficult to be motivated to do so. Jung emphasized the role dreams play in our development. Since the aneurysm, I have been unable to remember almost all of my dreams, so I can't analyze them.

At almost the two-year mark, after trying acupuncture and reading different Buddhist, Stoic, and other philosophical texts, one of the books I read was *The Doors of Perception* by Aldous Huxley. The book chronicles his experience experimenting with peyote. Now, I've avoided hallucinogens my entire life, however, there seemed to be something romantic about exploring this realm. Since my balance and vision were still not completely healed, I figured dabbling in pharmaceuticals such as these might be worthwhile.

I spoke with my consigliere, Mr. Mxyzptlk, named after the comic book imp who harasses Superman. He advised me to immediately participate in this scheme. However, my only problem, as he saw it, was where to acquire peyote. He raised a good point. I began to do some research and discovered The United States passed a law allowing the Native American Church to incorporate the use of peyote in their religious practices.

Upon doing further research, unfortunately, I discovered there are no Native American Churches nearby. So, I was back to square one. Although, I am hoping if the doors of perception stay closed, perhaps someone will open a window. I thought I could order peyote online, and I found a website for a distributor located in Holland. Then, of course, I imagined unwittingly participating in a sting operation in which a joint task force of DEA and FBI agents initiated a two-pronged attack on my domicile early in the morning. As the zip ties are cinched tight around my wrists and ankles, I can kiss due process goodbye as I am hauled off to some black site, wherein the words of Maynard from the film Charley Varrick, "They will go to work on me with a pair of pliers and a blowtorch." Therefore, I will probably avoid indulging in this fantasy of hallucinogens.

The other day, I participated in a zoom chat for a support group, and one of the case managers mentioned seeing Elvis play The Cow Palace in California. It had been toward the end of Elvis's career, but he still put on a phenomenal show. The more I thought about it, the more optimistic I became. Even though there's uncertainty, concerning my future, and I may not have the same goals/motivation as I did before, I will continue to heal and adjust. Elvis may not have been the same when he played The Cow Palace, but he still put on a good show.

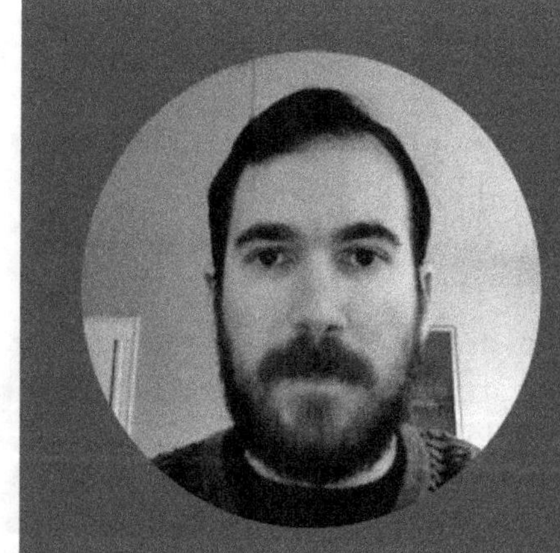

Meet Andrew Davie

Andrew Davie received an MFA in creative writing from Adelphi University. He taught English in Macau on a Fulbright Grant as well as other countries. In June of 2018, he survived a ruptured brain aneurysm and subarachnoid hemorrhage. His other writing and work can be found in links on his website: asdavie.wordpress.com

Story Callout:

Staying Safe During GLOBAL PANDEMIC

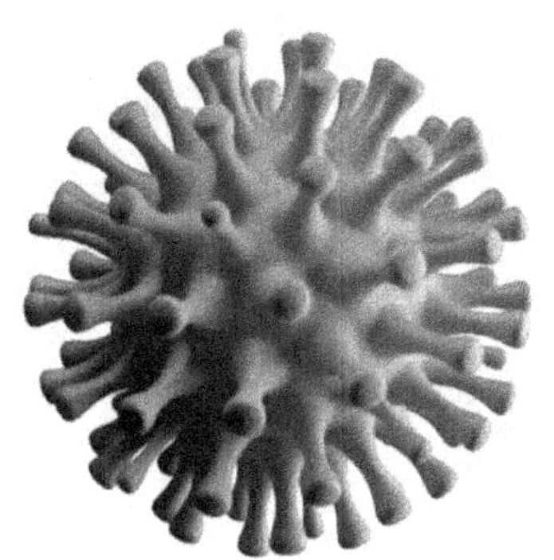

We are accepting stories for the Winter 2020 issue of HOPE Magazine about how you are staying safe during the pandemic.

These are challenging times indeed and your story can help others.

Our Winter 2020 issue of HOPE Magazine will be largely dedicated to this important topic.

Your Story has Value!

And now the details...

- We prefer an article length of 800-1,000 words. Longer or shorter pieces will be considered.
- When submitting, please include a photo or photos to be included with your piece.

Please email your submission to mystory@tbihopeandinspiration.com.

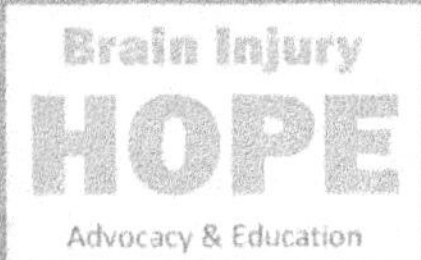

Brain Injury Meets Parenthood

By Sarah V. Jackson

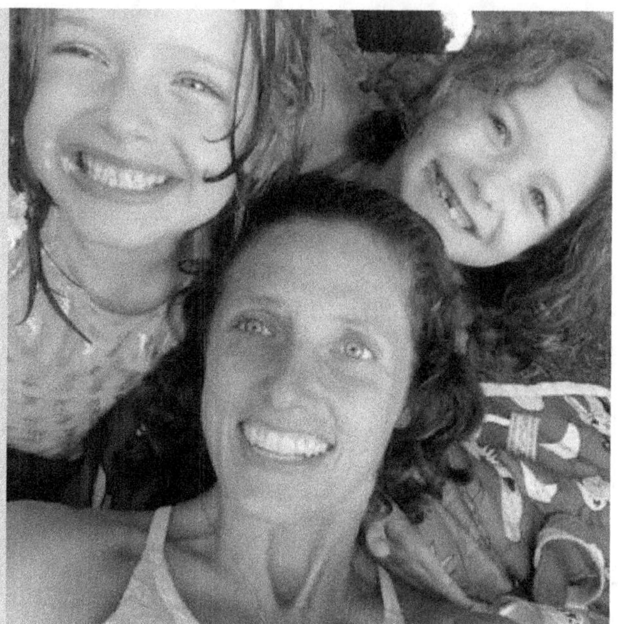

Since my head injury, or hospital stay, I will briefly, or humorously, discuss some of the issues that once stood in my way. More clearly, following written and verbal directions. Getting dressed in the morning was an issue. Having a list telling me what to do was, and still does, play a significant part in my daily living. Changing pants, shirts, undergarments, and shoes often got confused with which clothes I was going to wear that day and how I was going to initiate such tasks.

With the process of having to greet each day as a new day, greeting a new person, myself, with new limitations, I had the benefit of rediscovering myself every 24 hours, though the task gets tiring after a while. Having to reciprocate the same tasks on someone else though, like a kid for example, and the tasks becomes, *"Dress-yourself-or-stay-in-your-pajamas-and-I'll- carry-you-to-school-because-I'm-not-putting-up-with-your-attitude"* kind-of-day.

> *"I have become fairly comfortable with putting my orange juice in the microwave for thirty seconds each morning, so as to not scorch the nerves in my teeth."*

I have become fairly comfortable with putting my orange juice in the microwave for thirty seconds each morning, so as to not scorch the nerves in my teeth. Participating in my twice daily hygiene work-out sessions feels like I am participating in a triathlon consisting of toothbrushing, flossing and mouth washing and gum picking (when necessary) on a daily basis. I am sure to be a contender in the Winner's Circle for this event (I always knew I was an athlete).

Based on my oral hygiene expertise, I am fairly certain I can now dress myself before putting my shoes on, as opposed to after I put my shoes on. Easy-peazy, I say. I've got this routine down.

My kids, on the other hand, have no excuse. I used to follow written directions on how to perform such tasks until I had them etched in my memory and could perform them second-nature. My kids, however, are just wanting to remain kids and make my life miserable by refusing to do what I ask of them.

They have a list by the door saying what they need for school each day and it is their job to make sure they have required items.

Lesson #1: You have to want to get better. The desire to perform well, or to reach your optimum level, is in your bones. This goes for the injured or the child. When the child refuses to listen or is just playing a game to see if you remember to get on their case, it feels like you are simply filling space and your efforts become wasted. The saying goes, "You can lead a horse to water, but you can't make him drink." One can only try so hard before finally, the parent or caregiver, has to step back and say, "You have the tools, you know what's expected, good luck."

Tomorrow will be better, I say, as I watch my six-year-old strut out the door for school this morning. Not paying any attention to my Oh-So-Wonderful-Sign I have strategically placed in the doorway, or her snack that I put on the counter for her, or her unzipped backpack in the middle of the floor, or her extra bag of snow pants, boots, hats and gloves, '

I lower my head and shoulders to the floor with a sigh (far from relief) and shake my head. Surely, she will get better in time, but I can only try so hard. What is next on my list-of-things-to-do for the day?

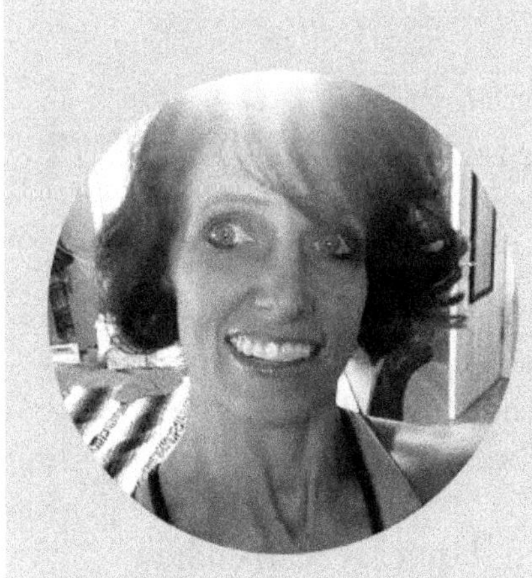

Meet Sarah V. Jackson

Sarah sustained a severe traumatic brain injury at the age of 15 after getting in a car with a underage drinking driver. She is the author of 'You're Getting Better Every Day.' After spreading her story to audiences nationwide, she is now a wife and mother of two girls. Read more about Sarah's story in her book and on her website www.sarahjspeaks.com as she continues to fight the battle of drinking and driving, underage drinking, poor choices and traumatic brain injury awareness.

Pandemics & Brain Injury

By Jen Dodge

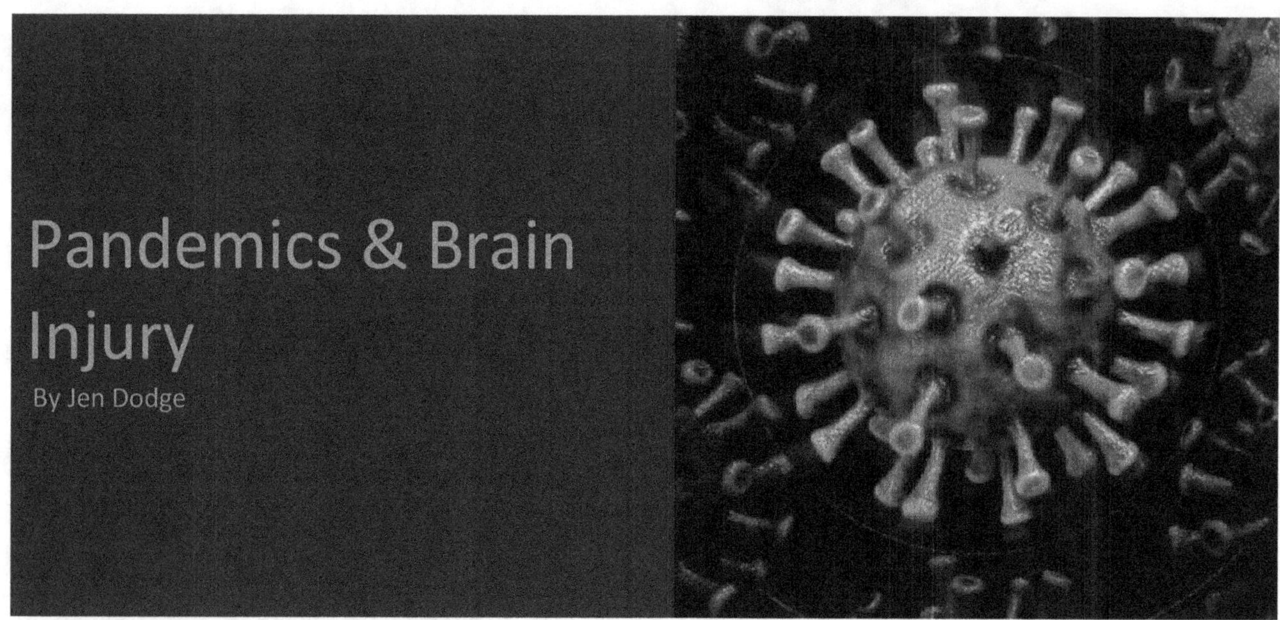

I was recently watching a clip that caught my attention and I want to start this by sharing some of their words. "Imagine one day you woke up in a foreign country. Everything looks similar but slightly different. You are not really sure how you got here. You certainly did not ask to come. And you wish you could just go home. Change is difficult for us all. Particularly when it happens suddenly, without warning. But for millions of Americans living with Traumatic Brain Injury, this is not the first time their lives have been turned upside down. And adapting once again to a 'new normal' may be especially challenging."

> *"Just when I thought living with a brain injury would be the hardest thing I would ever have to do, a pandemic entered the scene."*

Just when I thought living with a brain injury would be the hardest thing I would ever have to do, a pandemic entered the scene. One of the many things that makes living with a brain injury so difficult is the amount of mental energy needed to survive a day. That mental energy taxes an already exhausted, damaged brain. When you add a pandemic to the mix your daily mental energy needs go up 100 notches and your damaged brain suffers greatly.

With this pandemic I have lost my routine and five and a half years ago, I quickly learned how important routine was to living life with a TBI. My current routine is not natural; it is not intuitive.

• Stay six feet away from people (not just thinking it and remembering to do it, but actually having to calculate what six feet looks like is quite hard for me because I really struggle with visual spatial reasoning now).

• Wear a mask (remembering to pack it when I leave home, remembering to wear it when I enter a store, remembering to put it back on if I take it off to answer the phone at work or to catch my breath)

• Follow the arrows in the grocery stores (grocery shopping is so hard for my rattled brain [the noise, the stimulation, the chaos, following my grocery list, etc.] now add to it having to follow these arrows in the store for one-way traffic).

• The amount of stress I experience daily is now increased greatly with the worry of catching the virus, with the extra work that is required to live life, with the attitudes of people around you regarding the virus, and with trying to keep informed about the latest regarding Covid-19. Stress can really exacerbate TBI symptoms and I am feeling this effect daily.

• Social distancing from family and friends (living with a TBI is lonely as it is, now I'm forced to stay away from my already reduced social circle). The staying home part of this pandemic was actually easy for me as this was nothing new, but not seeing my friends was a little different and challenging at times.

Because I have lost my routine, because living during a pandemic requires more mental energy, because everything I do during this time is ten times harder than it was before, I feel like I'm back to my early days of my TBI. I require much more sleep, rest, and quiet time than I did before Covid-19 entered my world. This pandemic is taking a toll on me and my rattled brain, a toll that I fear will take a long time to recover from

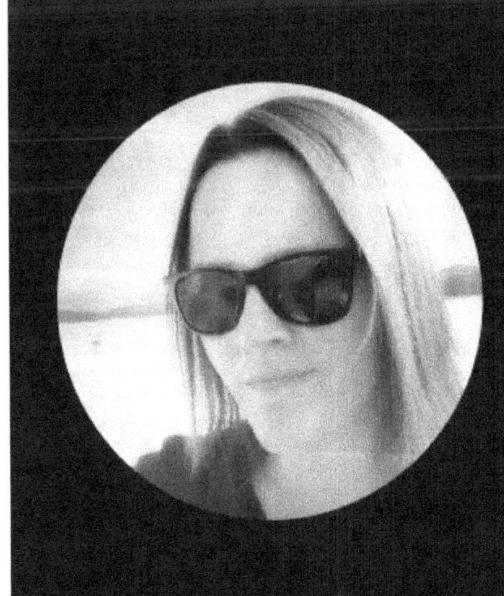

Meet Jen Dodge

Jen is a 37 year old resident of Northern New Hampshire. On August 19, 2014, she was hit by an SUV while riding her bicycle on a group ride. Since the accident she has written several articles titled "Confessions of a Concussed Cyclist" to help inform others and as a form of therapy for herself. She is a certified Special Education teacher, and an avid cyclist. Jen uses her own story to encourage people to become informed about the invisible disability of a brain injury and to be kind to cyclists and SHARE THE ROAD!

Discovering the New Molly

By Lyrsa Smith

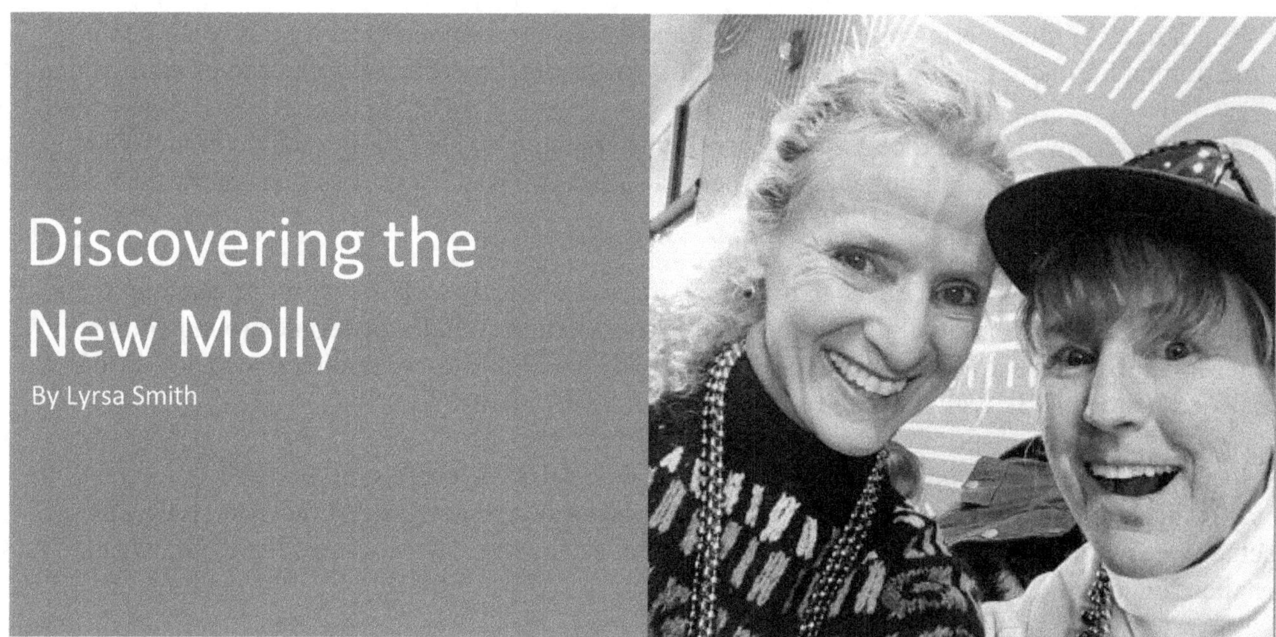

Stephen King, the renowned author who has scared us crazy with his horror stories, once described what frightens him most.

"I'm most afraid of losing my mind," he said. "You lose your identity, your sense of who you are, where you are."

I've witnessed the effects of seeing a loved one lose that sense of identity in a different way – through brain injury. And as her primary caregiver, I've watched how she's navigated the strange and frightening circumstances surrounding the Covid-19 pandemic.

"It is terrifying to lose your personality, your ability to reason and regulate your emotions, to lose your life as you'd built it and knew it, to lose your place in the world."

My older sister, Molly has a severe brain injury from carbon monoxide poisoning, an accident that occurred in a hotel 25 years ago. Her husband, Walt, died at her side from CO poisoning. It was a nightmare. It is terrifying to lose your personality, your ability to reason and regulate your emotions, to lose your life as you'd built it and knew it, to lose your place in the world.

Molly has made impressive adjustments over the decades. She's gone up and down, backwards and forward. Without a doubt, though, she is not who she used to be. As Stephen King fears, Molly lost her identity, where she was in life, and much of who she was. She is a different person and she carries on.

For me and Molly's other family members, we discover who the new Molly is on any given day, and we do not guess who she will be tomorrow. I used to say that I redefine normal every day. More recently, I've stopped defining what normal is at all.

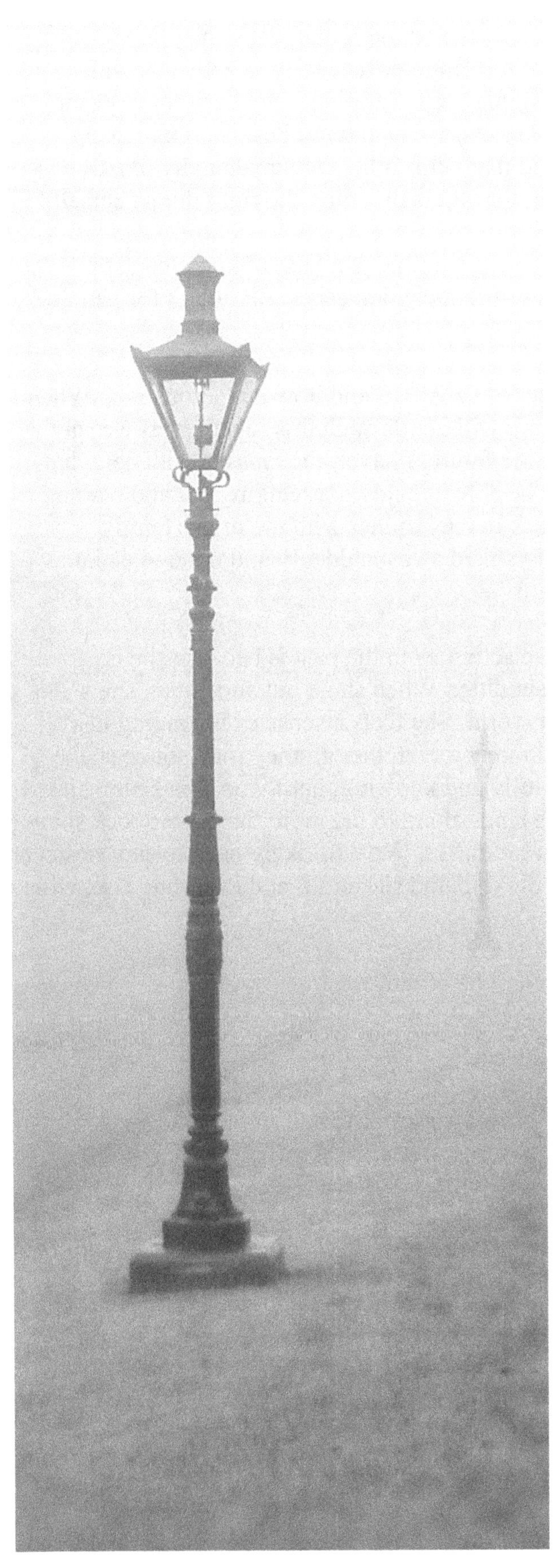

Stephen King wrote a book that many people these days feel like they're living in. King's novel *The Stand* is about a viral pandemic, a particular strain of influenza, no less, that decimates most of the world's population.

Sound familiar? In these difficult days of Covid-19, there's a lot to be afraid of. Most of us know enough to be fearful and concerned and yet, not enough to know how to fully protect ourselves or our loved ones. Most of us feel some anxiety. We don't know what tomorrow will be like.

We're adjusting to our new lifestyles of staying home, physically distancing, working from our kitchen tables, and keeping our social contact with others from the heart – and remote.

Molly lives about 20 miles from me in a residential home with four other people who each have a brain injury. They are under strict lockdown, as are the other supportive, assisted, and nursing care facilities in Colorado. Molly has her own bedroom with large windows. She and her housemates share several bathrooms and some common areas, including a big comfy living room, a kitchen, and dining room. She stays six feet away and mostly spends her time in her room reading, listening to music, and watching TV or movies.

Her residence is staffed 24/7 by professionals, heroes who come and go on eight-hour shifts. They care for Molly and her housemates by preparing meals, delivering medications, and providing watchfulness, company, and comfort. Everyone is very careful.

About once a week, I go to the house wearing my mask to deliver medicines, toothpaste or other items Molly needs, and a large Frappuccino from the take-out window of the nearby Starbucks. I leave everything at the front door, and I step into the yard as a masked staff person collects the bag. I can see Molly in the living room, and we wave to each other and give the ASL sign for "I love you."

Molly is being a real trouper. Like all of us, she's missing connection in the ways she prefers. Hugs from her family members, close greetings with friends, and laughter face to face with acquaintances. She's following the rules and is doing pretty well managing her frustration – not easy for a person with a brain injury even in non-Covid-19 times. I call her every day and my best encouragement strategy is to remind her that she's keeping healthy, and that helps others to stay healthy too. She seems to appreciate having the larger mission of caring for others by doing the right things herself.

Most of us are experiencing various levels of confusion and fear due to a lack of knowledge or answers about Covid-19. These emotions and realities of life today are especially tough for people with brain injuries.

It's hard for Molly to understand the widespread impact of Covid-19 and how dangerous it is. When I speak with her, I try to provide a hopeful outlook that we will get through this together, as we stay apart. I try to raise her spirits and keep her focused on the future. I haven't discussed with her what that future may be like. I don't know when or if she'll be able to enjoy her hanging out and reading time at Starbucks, her manicure and pedicure treatments, having dinner with me or her family members at her favorite bustling restaurants. It was all yanked away suddenly and none of us know when or if we can settle into those social comforts again.

I know that the primary reason Molly has enjoyed these activities in the past is because she is surrounded by other people, side by side, shoulder to shoulder. When she's out and about, she's engages as best she can and she feels part of the larger world. She feels a sense of belonging in a crowd of people who don't know she has a severe brain injury even though they may notice she's different somehow. I'm looking forward to hugging Molly and knowing that I won't make her sick. I want to have her in the passenger seat of my car as she sings along to the radio the classic rock songs she loves. When that day comes, we may both be wearing masks. We will likely need to stay six feet apart from everyone we encounter. It will be a changed world and she and I, and everyone else, will be leading changed lives.

And yet, I believe Molly has made up her mind. She won't be afraid.

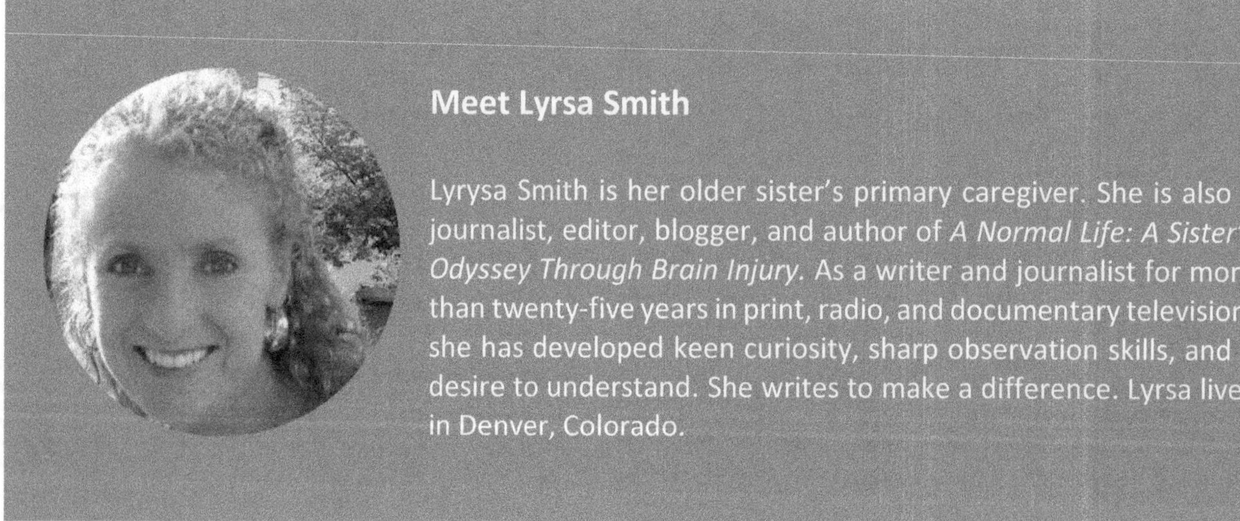

Meet Lyrsa Smith

Lyrysa Smith is her older sister's primary caregiver. She is also a journalist, editor, blogger, and author of *A Normal Life: A Sister's Odyssey Through Brain Injury.* As a writer and journalist for more than twenty-five years in print, radio, and documentary television, she has developed keen curiosity, sharp observation skills, and a desire to understand. She writes to make a difference. Lyrsa lives in Denver, Colorado.

Not an Island

By Eddie Conrardy

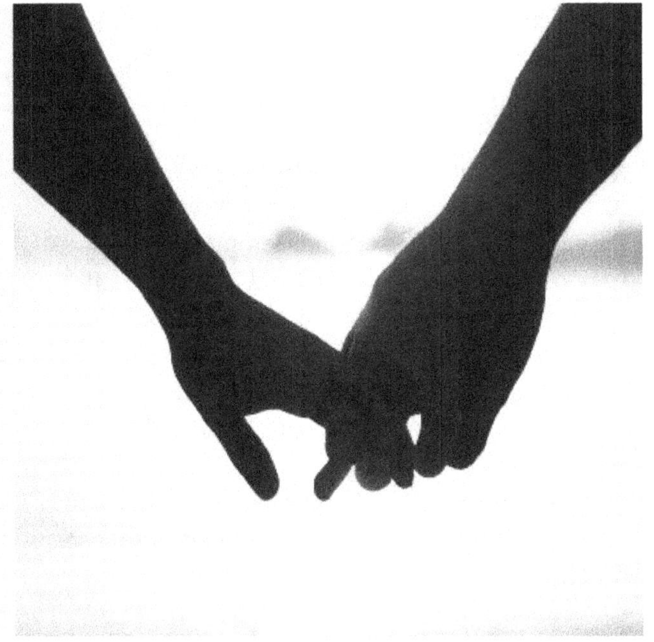

COVID-19. Global pandemic. Social distancing. Lockdowns. Everyone has essentially become an island unto themselves. Have we been affected by any of this? I don't expect it's anything too different than most people are dealing with: kids finishing school at home, not going in to work, limited outings, marveling at the obsession so many people had with toilet paper, or a kid's birthday without friends. That one was rough.

Smack in the middle of all this, my wife and I celebrated our twenty-third wedding anniversary. We had many pre-TBI years together, and our first twenty years I would describe as fairly typical. We worked, traveled, had kids, and we really enjoyed life.

Then, following an accident in 2017 that resulted in a severe TBI, these last three years for my wife as a TBI survivor and for me as her caregiver have been much different. We are still learning to adjust to many difficulties in almost every aspect of our lives. Then there's the myriad issues the pandemic and subsequent lockdowns brought. Funny enough, the issues of the last few months have not been particularly disrupting for either of us.

"We had many pre-TBI years together, and our first twenty years I would describe as fairly typical. We worked, traveled, had kids, and we really enjoyed life."

It was difficult to manage any social gatherings or recreational outings before COVID-19, but it's something we've dealt with together as a family. Living through the pandemic has mostly been continuing the new normal of life for us.

"Normal" being very much a relative term for TBI survivors and their families.

Regarding our recent anniversary, with things being what they are right now, it was a low-key celebration at home. My grand visions of recreating our first date couldn't have happened anyway, as that particular Bennigan's restaurant has long since closed. I have to say though, they had the best artery-hardening Monte Cristos! I suppose we could have watched the same movie we did on that night long ago, but she can no longer sit through an entire movie. To be fair, I'm not sure I could sit through the entirety of "Barbarian Queen" now, either.

Instead, I took my wife on a photographic tour of our wedding and first few years together. She remembered quite a bit. Some things she even started talking about before we got to the pictures. There were still hazy areas, especially the time around the years 1999-2000 and onward. The gaps in her memories are very pronounced. We had fun looking through all the photos, recalling various stories, relating memories that have been forgotten, and reflecting.

The events of the past the years - and the past few months - have certainly been cause for reflection on many things.

One of the more important truths that has been made abundantly clear to me in this time is that no man is an island. It is equally true that no couple and no family is an island. We are here and together thanks in no small part to the incredible family and friends we have. They are all very much a part of us and who we are, and I cannot thank them enough for being part of our lives.

I know not everyone is fortunate enough to have this kind of support as a TBI survivor or caregiver, and the situation is made even more difficult in these recent months with trying to navigate social distancing and lockdowns.

'No Man is an Island'
-John Donne, 1624

No man is an island, entire of itself;
every man is a piece of the continent,
a part of the main.

If a clod be washed away by the sea,
Europe is the less,
as well as if a promontory were,
as well as any manner of thy friends
or of thine own were.

Any man's death diminishes me,
because I am involved in mankind.
And therefore never send to know
for whom the bell tolls;
it tolls for thee.

It is easy to see why so many of us in this situation feel like we are in it alone, that we are indeed islands. Just remember that there are no awards for trying to do everything alone.

Every situation, every person, and every TBI is unique. Offering advice is tricky in even the simplest of situations, so consider the following an observation on what has helped me.

Let others into your life - the good, the bad, the struggles, and the victories. It is not always an easy thing. As an introvert, believe me I know. Do not ignore or rebuff offers of support. Do the opposite by making an effort to seek it out, even if it's only for casual conversation and a sense of normalcy. Maybe you do not need a lot of support or help at the moment, but eventually we all do. And when you reach that point, you'll have already done what I consider the hard part, being vulnerable.

Whether you are a survivor or caregiver, invite those around you over to the island. Hopefully, you'll discover that you're not an island after all.

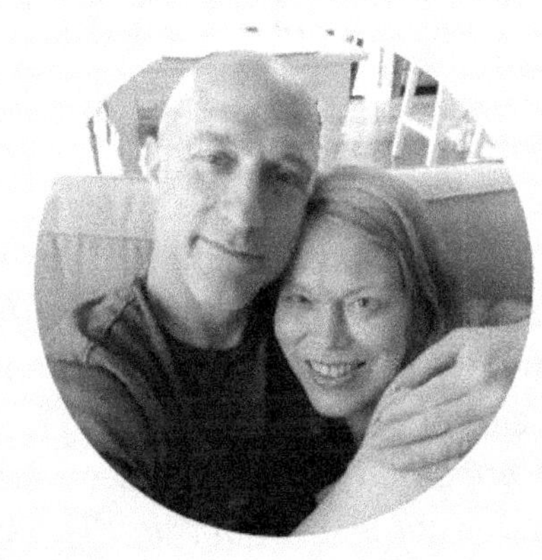

Meet Eddie Conrardy

After nearly three years, Eddie still struggles with the changes that those three little letters (TBI) have wrought for his wife and family. As husband, father, and caregiver he does his best to manage it all - and gently reminds himself from time to time that he's not an island.

"Love recognizes no barriers. It jumps hurdles, leaps fences, penetrates walls to arrive at its destination full of hope."

— Maya Angelou

Brain Quake

By Roman Ponomarchuks

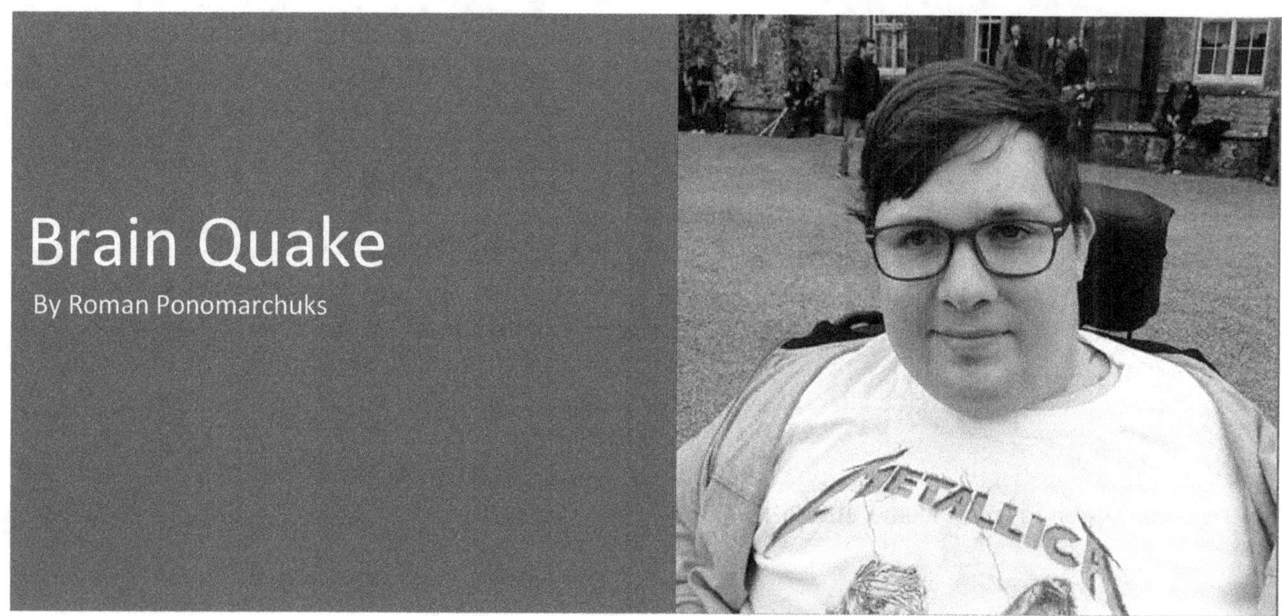

Brain Quake

Mistakes are easy.
Learning from them
When I'm falling through
My disposable life
Into eternal emptiness
So lonely
So separate
So hard to be friends
With myself when I always land
In the same
Black fortress
Is the hard part.

Meet Roman Ponomarchuks

Roman is a thirty-three year old man living in Ireland. He recovering from a 2014 road traffic accident in which he lost the use of his arms and legs. He started dictating poems a year ago and hopes they bring hope and inspiration to others. He lives in a residential institution, and knows that these gifts can often be in short supply. He hopes to publish a book of his poetry in the coming months, entitled, "My Best Enemy Is Myself."

"Courage is resistance to fear, mastery of fear - not absence of fear."

— Mark Twain

Drastic Changes Again

By James Scott

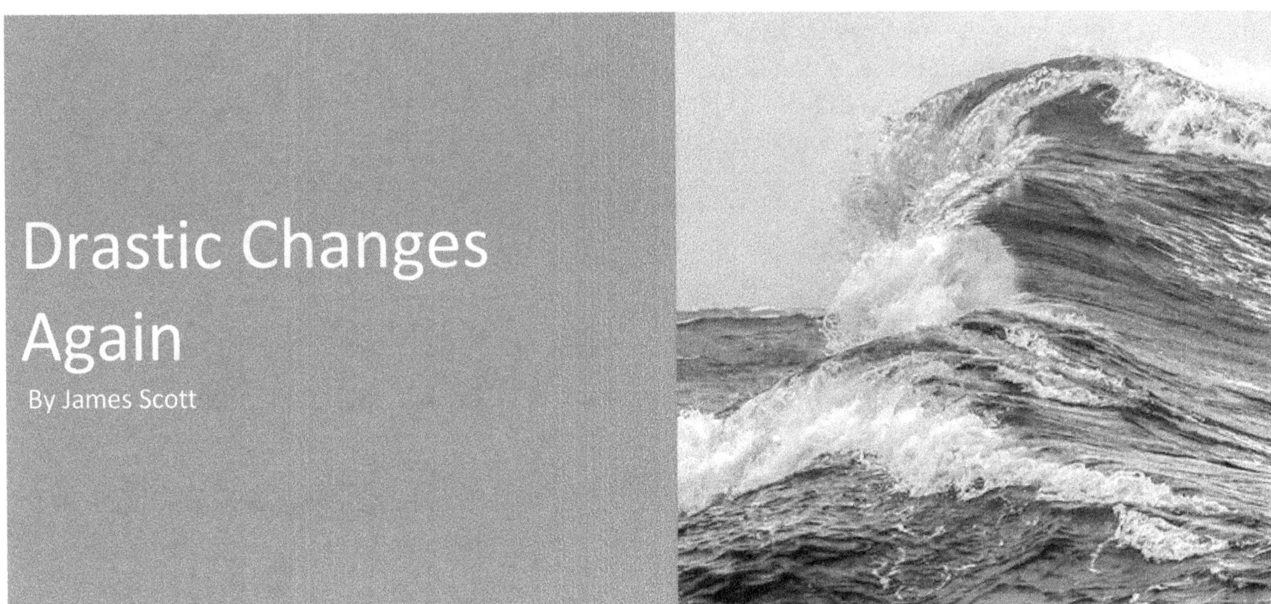

I recently was honored to have a piece I wrote on acceptance featured in the Spring 2020 issue of *Hope Magazine.* In my writing I tried to express my deep gratitude for all the amazing help I have received throughout my recovery from a car crash on 7/4/06. In the short time since I wrote *Living Life on Life's Terms,* something I never thought would happen has occurred: Another drastic change. Only this time it is the way the world functions around me, not the way I function in the world that has changed. Call it a pandemic, national emergency, call it whatever you prefer, but the bottom line is that a lot of us have seen huge change in our daily lives.

Over the course of one's life, the only thing that seems to be constant or guaranteed is change. These transition periods, although a constant in life, can be distressing. While not necessarily limited to negative changes like loss or illness, these difficult periods, even after positive developments, can certainly be challenging.

> *"Since my injury, I've felt an eerie calm from an expectation that after the crash, I would be insulated from additional traumatic events, or at least better prepared."*

When we talk about loss, the first thing that comes to mind is death. Death is of course the ultimate loss, a singular event from which there is no possible return to a prior state. As I always like to say when I feel like I'm pontificating, I can only offer my personal experience, although perhaps readers will relate. Since my injury, I've felt an eerie calm from an expectation that after the crash, I would be insulated from additional traumatic events, or at least better prepared. Not that I would be immune from all the ills of ordinary humanism or never experience tragedy again, rather my handling of the situation would be exemplary.

In case you are wondering, this hunch has been proven inaccurate by the unease I've experienced living through this period. Don't get me wrong, I'm blessed that my friends and family are healthy and that I still have a job, but at the same time, the sudden change in the ways of the world has thrown me for a loop. As much as I try to remain positive and remind myself that "this too shall pass," the cunning trap of self-centered based pity is right at my doorstep during this period.

In my now over ten years as a member of the Krempels Center, a day program for the brain in jury community, among the many helpful tools I have acquired is the ability to identify faulty thinking. While I don't have the complete list of these logical errors or mistakes in thinking, common enough to have a fancy name, memorized, I poignantly remember one such error as being personalization. Perhaps I strongly identified with this particular error because I had perfected making it.

After my brain injury, there was a period where my world became quite small and hyper focused on me. Early therapy was focused on assessing skills, identifying deficits, setting goals, and charting the progress I made. Often an unintended consequence of this intense period of reflection and analysis is the tendency to see the world as revolving around yourself. I have found that it takes work and a constant effort to break free of this mindset and simply join the stream of life.

To join the stream of life, to be another functioning part of the world, isn't that what I worked so hard in all those rehab sessions for? Maybe, but it is not always an easy role to slide back into regardless of the progress made and time passed. I hate making assumptions, but I have to think that any surprise that shakes the norms of the entire world such as this global pandemic causes widespread unease. Add to that the personal past experience of having our lives derailed for brain injury survivors and it's no wonder that these may be stressful times.

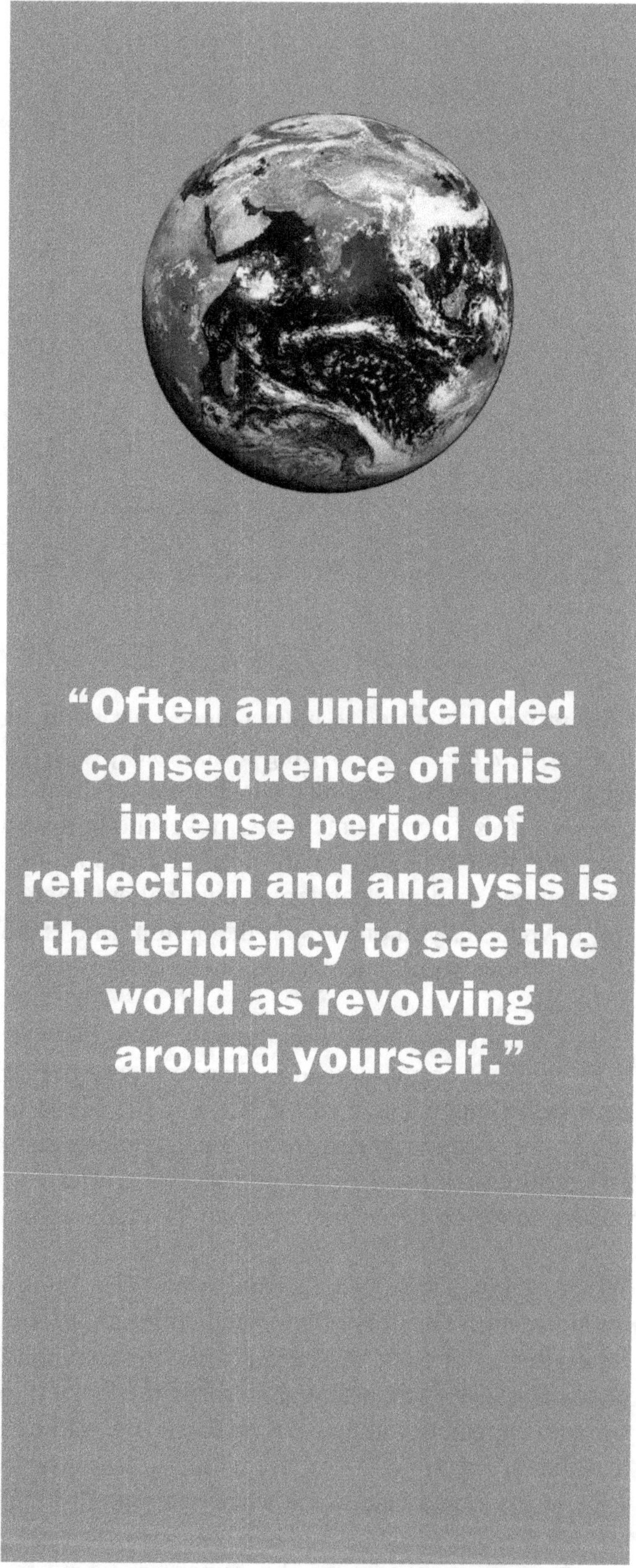

Perhaps the most beneficial aspect of joining an amazing community-based day program like Krempels' Center is being a member of a group of survivors striving towards creating a new life after brain injury! None of us members are happy about the injury that made us eligible for membership, but Krempels' is an absolute blessing in our lives.

Like any transition, learning to and becoming comfortable with life with a brain injury can be challenging: At the Center, we accept each other where we are at in our journeys, sharing experience and strength through the telling of our stories. I cannot help but see the parallels with the current global crisis and the need for feeling a part of a community that all of us have.

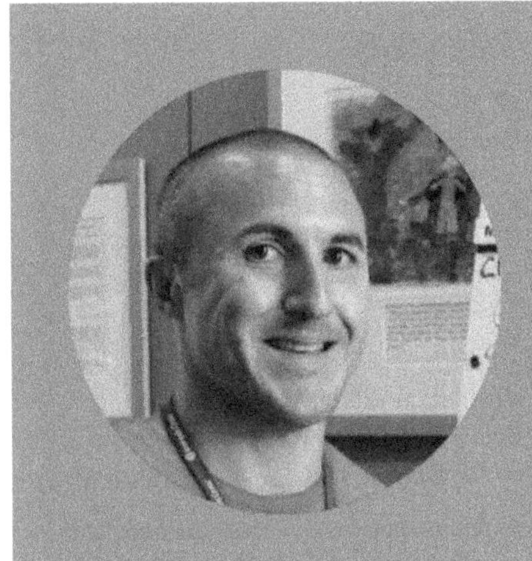

Meet James Scott

James sustained a TBI in a motor vehicle crash in July of 2006. Recognizing the cautionary value in his personal story, Jim first began speaking to students with KC's Community Education program. Jim has also worked with Northeast Rehabilitation Hospital's Think First National Injury Prevention Foundation. In 2012, Jim published a memoir titled More Than a Speed Bump: Life Before and After Traumatic Brain Injury.

Living With Hope

By Patrick Brigham

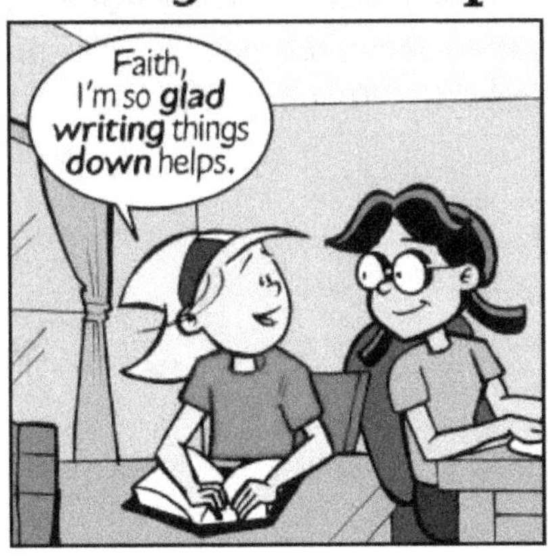

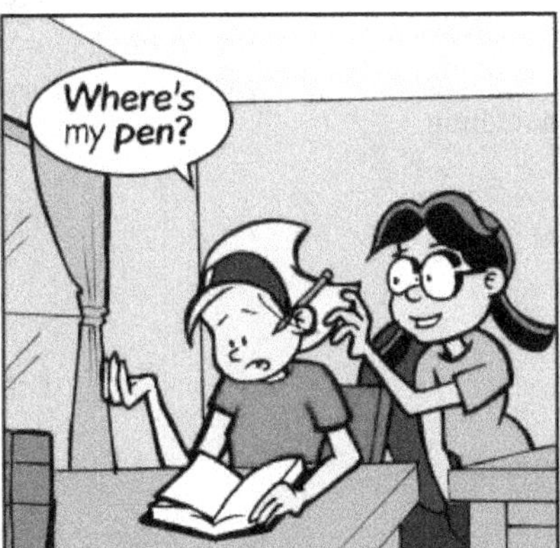

Introductions

By Rebecca Veenstra

My new self?
I'm confused.
My new self?
Whatever for?

The old one was fine
Far as I could tell
Probably coulda used
some tinkering in truth

But it was still going down the road just fine
What do they say?
If it ain't broke don't fix it?

Now that it's broken tho?
All Humpty Dumpty style

Swallowed by quicksand in the road
Where they found me
Irretrievably lost
Like it was never there
An entire self...gone
Just like that

It must be replaced with something no?
My new self...of course...this makes some sense now.
Reluctantly...I ask for the mantle...I'll wear it, yes...

Oh? I am wearing it?
What d'ya know...

I have been? For how long??
Since they found me? You don't say...

Awkward...ok...um. Well if ya don't mind making
introductions

I'm afraid we are not acquainted

This self and I are perfect strangers,
Though we have been tethered

Since I woke up in the road that was like quicksand
swallowing the thing that I called my life.

Meet Rebecca Veenstra

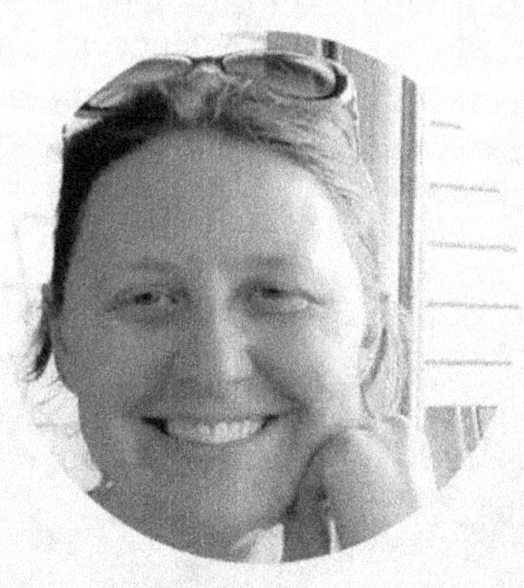

Rebecca writes...

"I am 47 years old. I was an herbalist, runner, work out fanatic, health food nut and writer before a run in with a dump truck in 2014 changed my life forever. I live in Northern Michigan with my two Chihuahuas.

I enjoy gardening and photography. This is my first piece of writing since the crash. It feels good to have my words back again. I am beginning to think of ways I can pay back all the kindness and caring I received through my recovery. I hope to someday find a path that gives me the opportunity to advocate for and support others with TBI and PTSD."

High Functioning

By Thomas Sanders

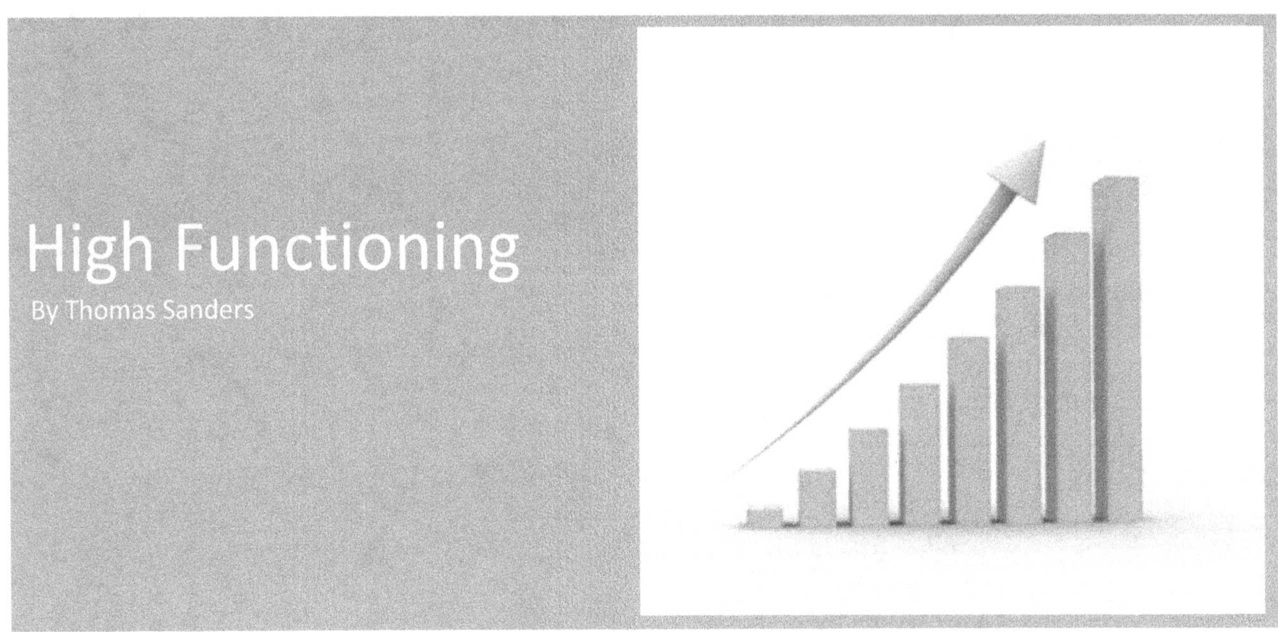

I am a success story. Apparently.

Nearly twenty years later, I am homeowner with an active social life and a steady federal job in Washington, DC. I have been fired from other jobs. I make excuses every time. *The business was relocating, that's the only reason. I was one of many who got laid off, that's the only reason. I wasn't actually calling her a name, not really.*

But I'm OK now. Usually. You might not like me when I am mad. I don't. I am reassured by the job security of my current federal position that I earned nine years ago with a non-competitive placement, because I have a letter from the DC Government Department of Human Service that sheepishly concedes I am "severely disabled and therefore eligible for a Schedule A Placement."

> *I have a letter from the DC Government Department of Human Service that sheepishly concedes I am "severely disabled and therefore eligible for a Schedule A Placement."*

I'm not sure I agree with that "severely" label. It sure feels insulting. But I am not very good at my job. This is unimaginably frustrating because in a previous life, nearly twenty years ago, I believe I was a very intelligent person. I am *supposed* to be smart.

Then a week before I was set to begin classes for my junior year of college in Atlanta, I visited friends in Southern California. The first couple days of the trip, the only ones I would remember, were wonderful.

But my friends and I felt young and invincible, our car was traveling way too fast, we crashed, and that life concluded.

My vaguest memories would begin a few weeks and three hospitals later in Washington, where my parents had moved from my hometown of Minneapolis, Minnesota, less than a year ago.

One tricky bit at work, with a traumatic brain injury, is that "intelligence" is not a simple, single metric. And I'll argue that parts of my damaged brain still excel. But when your short-term memory proves on a daily basis to be far too short term, the ballgame is effectively over.

I have long grown used to the frustration of reciprocating "hello" at the office when a face I swear I've never seen greets me by name in the corridor.

Yes, you can set calendar reminders on your work computer, and I do. Yes, you can take a notepad and a pen with you every time you report to coworkers' offices, and I do (sometimes I forget). Yes, you can "decorate" your own office with Post-It reminders, and I do.

They say the devil is in the details, and appropriately enough it feels like the most common qualification found in any job description is "attention to detail." Unfortunately, this often feels like my single worst attribute now. Any task or interaction at the workplace--or the world--includes many interacting, moving pieces. Meanwhile, I cherish the routine. Not the mundane, mind you, but the actual routine.

Nobody wants to relate to a stereotypical, cliched autistic kid who is terrified of change. I will comfortably, efficiently, and accurately perform the task I know.

But every job consists of a perpetually evolving series of duties, and so I'm not very good at mine. Strangely, I believe many of my coworkers do not realize.

I am a high-functioning idiot and like to think I cover it well most of the time. After all, so long as I have been given specific instructions, preferably very recently, ideally detailed in an email to reference, I will do what you want. Quickly and correctly.

But then I'll direct a document to the wrong place.

"Thomas, we just talked about this. Yesterday. We changed that procedure. Now congressional letters about that topic are sent to this agency. You seriously don't remember our conversation?"

"No, no, yeah, yeah, that's right, I'll fix it."

And I do. And all things considered, my position is sufficiently low-level that my annual evaluations remain consistently better than average. Years ago I reached the top of the relatively modest pay ladder for my job and sure, I'd like to find a better one. Some colleagues and bosses understand my frustration at the dead-end nature of my unthinking position, and they pass along higher-paying job announcements that sound good for me, and encourage me to apply.

I usually do and maybe once a year I'll even be contacted for an interview, where I do my best to enunciate slowly, and present myself as the normal person I feign to be. One thing I do not tell anybody about, after I do not get one of these positions, is the palpable relief I feel to be remaining at the current job that I complain about. The one I know.

Because I do not actually trust myself to manage a more difficult position. Most of these job descriptions include "attention to detail," and it is very embarrassing to have such a steep learning curve. What happens when I can't cover it up at the next place?

But I am a success story. Apparently.

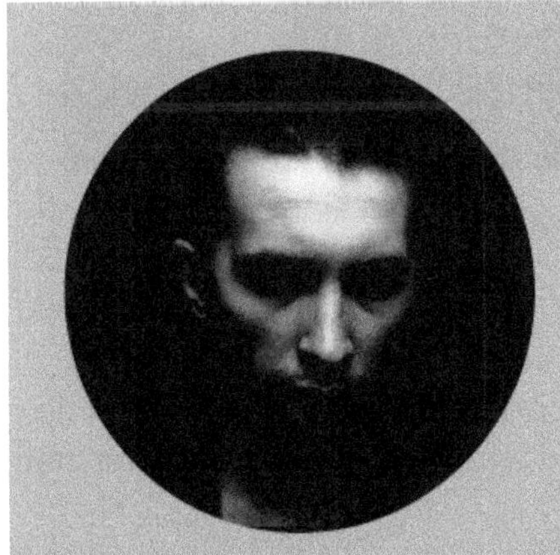

Meet Thomas Sanders

Thomas Sanders is, like so many District of Columbia residents, an employee of the federal government. After suffering a traumatic brain injury, he completed college and earned an MFA in Writing from Southampton College, and he has worked in New York City, South Florida, Costa Rica, and Washington, DC.

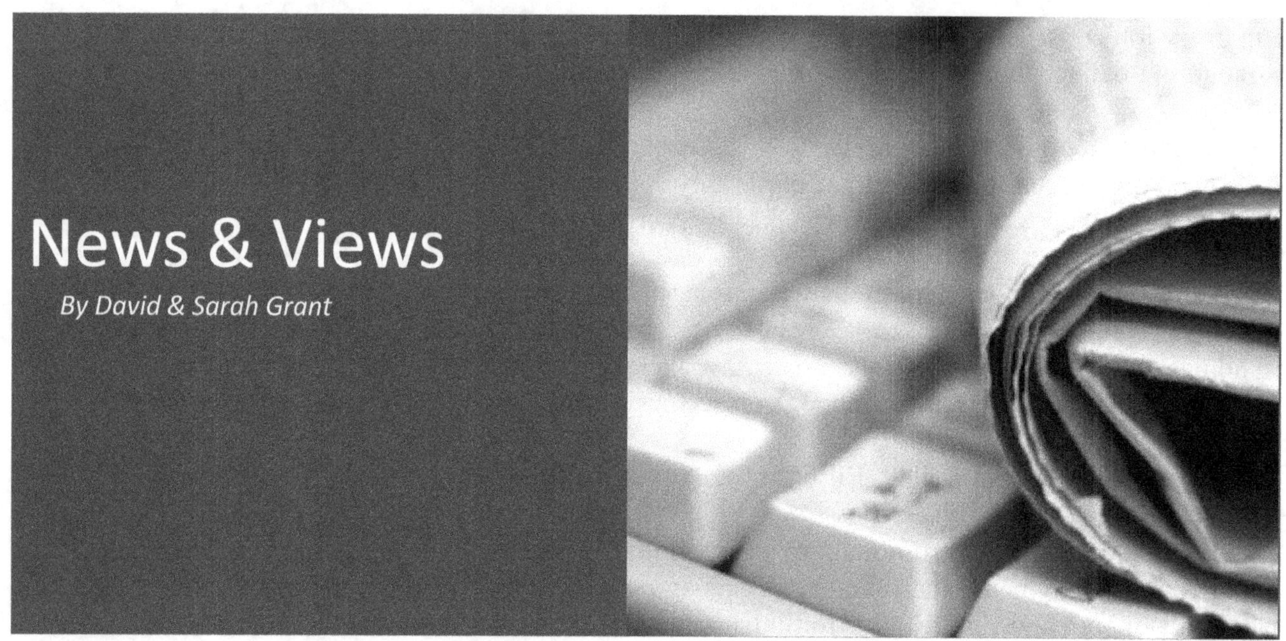

Hope Magazine has become the leading publication of the brain injury community. Now read in over sixty countries around the globe, every issue is very much like the one that you just read. We remain a vibrant, alive, (and at times vocal) voice for the brain injury community.

This past issue, typical of all prior issues, touches on current day events, brain injury challenges, and of course, solutions that have helped so many others to navigate the waters of life after *"everything changed."* This issue has more than passing reference to the COVID-19 pandemic.

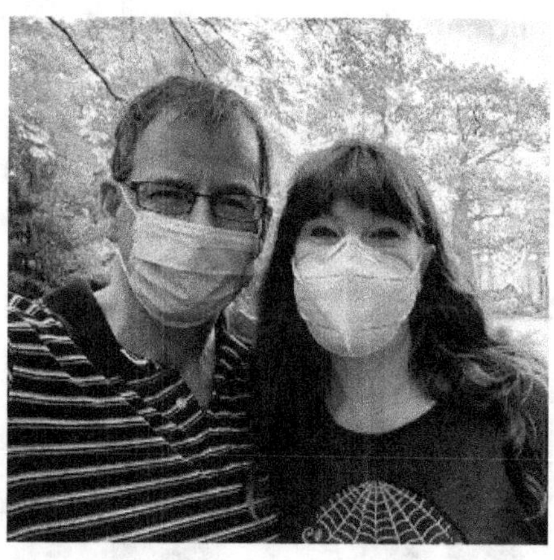

While brain injury is singularly the biggest challenge that most will ever face in their lifetimes, we are in the midst of a generational challenge – the global pandemic. In deciding to again ask for more stories about how you all are faring during the pandemic, it came back to one point – so many are struggling, and to gloss over this once-in-a-lifetime global challenge would be to disserve our readership.

As a community-supported publication, we could use your support. Like most of our issues, you'll not see any advertisers. We rely almost entirely on the generosity of our readers to help offset the expenses that come with publication. If you would like to help support HOPE Magazine, you can do so at www.tbihopeandinspiration.com/donation.html. If you do chose to help, a genuine and heartfelt thank you.

Peace.

~David & Sarah

www.ingramcontent.com/pod-product-compliance
Lightning Source LLC
Chambersburg PA
CBHW081256250726

48654CB00012B/1630